Carpal Tunnel Syndrome:
A Guide to Daily Activities

Occupational Therapy:
Skills for the Job of Living

Developed by

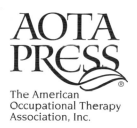

The American
Occupational Therapy
Association, Inc.

Introduction

Managing carpal tunnel syndrome can take time and patience. This syndrome of the hand and wrist can affect the basic activities of your daily life—how you work, do household tasks, and enjoy leisure time. As you recover, your occupational therapist and occupational therapy assistant will help you learn the safest ways to do daily activities.

This guide is a tool that you and your occupational therapist or occupational therapy assistant can use during and after your therapy sessions. This guide discusses:

- the causes, symptoms, and diagnosis of carpal tunnel syndrome;

- ways to manage carpal tunnel syndrome;

- advice for doing daily work, household, and leisure activities;

- exercises that may help prevent or reduce your symptoms; and

- general safety tips.

This guide refers to two different types of practitioners: occupational therapists and occupational therapy assistants. Occupational therapy assistants work under the supervision of occupational therapists. You may meet both types of practitioners during your treatment.

An occupational therapist will evaluate you, prepare your treatment plan, and may work with you during your therapy sessions. In many settings, an occupational therapy assistant, under the supervision of an occupational therapist, will carry out the treatment plan and work with you in your therapy.

Using This Guide

You and your occupational therapist or occupational therapy assistant will determine the best way to perform your daily activities. This guide includes many of the activities you will discuss.

Listen carefully and write any special instructions your occupational therapist, occupational therapy assistant, or doctor tells you in this guide. Ask questions if you're confused or if an activity that's important to you is not covered in this guide.

Remember: Your occupational therapist or occupational therapy assistant may change some of these instructions to reflect your individual needs. For example, he or she may suggest other ways to do the exercises shown in this booklet.

Throughout this guide, you will find references to splints and adapted or specially designed tools. Your occupational therapist or occupational therapy assistant will offer needed items or will give you information about where you can obtain them.

To learn more about occupational therapy, visit the American Occupational Therapy Association's Web site at www.aota.org or call 301-652-AOTA (2682).

Information to Remember

Occupational therapist's or occupational therapy assistant's name

Occupational therapist's or occupational therapy assistant's telephone number

Facility

Doctor's or hand surgeon's name and telephone number

Facility

About Carpal Tunnel Syndrome

Carpal tunnel syndrome is a common, painful condition that results from overuse of one's wrist or hand, from injury, or from other health problems. Although the syndrome is disabling for some people, it can be managed effectively with expert therapy and treatment.

Carpal tunnel syndrome is more common in women than in men, and it usually begins between the ages of 30 and 50. Grocery store checkers, accountants, musicians, meat packers, assembly line workers, and workers who use vibrating tools are more likely to develop the syndrome. Hobbies and activities like needlework, woodworking, gardening, and cleaning can contribute to carpal tunnel syndrome, as well. People who use computers for many hours a day may also develop this syndrome.

People with certain physical conditions also have a greater chance of developing carpal tunnel syndrome. These conditions include diabetes, rheumatoid arthritis, thyroid gland problems, obesity, and broken or dislocated wrist bones. In addition, the syndrome can arise during pregnancy, during menopause, or with contraceptive pill use.

Proper positioning of the hand and wrist, exercise, and frequent rest from repetitive activities can help prevent or reduce the symptoms of carpal tunnel syndrome.

Causes of Carpal Tunnel Syndrome

To understand carpal tunnel syndrome, it is helpful to look at the moving parts of the wrist.

The eight carpal bones and a strong ligament form a tunnel-like pathway in the wrist. The median nerve and nine flexor tendons run through this tunnel. The median nerve runs from the forearm into the hand. It provides feeling in the thumb and fingers and controls some of the thumb muscles. The flexor tendons control finger and thumb movement.

Normally, use of the hand does not cause problems. However, inflammation, swelling, or scarring may narrow the space next to the median nerve, and pinch or damage the median nerve. This pinching or damage may cause the symptoms of carpal tunnel syndrome.

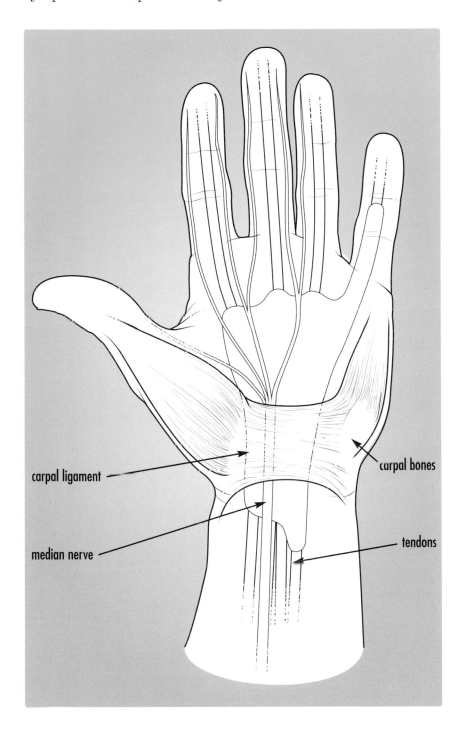

carpal ligament

carpal bones

median nerve

tendons

Symptoms

Symptoms of carpal tunnel syndrome may include:

- pain, burning, and a "pins and needles" feeling in the wrist and hand, especially in the thumb, index, and middle fingers;
- increased pain and tingling at night;
- problems gripping or making a fist;
- clumsiness when doing simple tasks like tying one's shoes or picking up small objects;
- a feeling that the fingers are swollen; and
- not being able to feel the difference between hot and cold.

Diagnosis

To find out if you have carpal tunnel syndrome, your doctor will do a physical examination and may do a simple nerve test called a nerve conduction study.

It is also helpful to write down your symptoms and share the information with your doctor. This information will help the doctor decide the best way to evaluate and treat your condition. Make detailed notes about:

- what symptoms you feel;
- where on your hand, wrist, or arm the symptoms occur;
- how long you have felt the symptoms;
- when you usually feel the symptoms; and
- what kinds of tasks, activities, or positions seem to cause the symptoms.

Carpal tunnel syndrome should be carefully evaluated because many nerve problems can mimic its symptoms. Likewise, carpal tunnel syndrome can mimic the symptoms of other hand and arm problems.

Managing Carpal Tunnel Syndrome

Carpal tunnel syndrome can be managed effectively with therapy, especially when therapy begins in the early stages of the syndrome. Surgery may be needed if other treatments do not work or if the syndrome is diagnosed in the late stages. If surgery is needed, your doctor may recommend rehabilitation, including occupational therapy, after the surgery.

Occupational therapy practitioners can:

- help evaluate and treat the condition, and provide ongoing analysis of the problem;
- correct the condition with splinting, therapy, ergonomic education, and lifestyle changes;
- improve the condition of the hand; and
- enhance the outcome of surgery if it is needed.

As described below, your occupational therapy program may include:

- management of swelling;
- use of a splint;
- use of adapted or specially designed tools; and
- exercise.

Your doctor may also suggest that you use medications. If other treatments are unsuccessful, surgery may be recommended.

Edema (Swelling) Management

If you have carpal tunnel syndrome and your hand is not moved or is immobilized, fluids may pool. As a result, you may develop edema, or swelling, in your hand, wrist, or arm. It is important to manage edema early to prevent severe problems.

Swelling in and around the joints can prevent normal motion. If normal motion is not restored, pooled fluids can cause continued, harmful tissue changes. This leads to a cycle that can be difficult to correct. Therefore, your joints usually should be allowed to move freely to improve blood circulation and prevent pooling of fluids.

To prevent or reduce swelling:

- Elevate your hand without tightly bending your elbow. Rest your hand on a pillow to your side, on a couch arm, on a car seat, or on someone else's shoulder.
- When elevating your hand, keep your hand above your elbow and keep your elbow above your shoulder.
- Comfortably open and close your hand into a comfortable fist or partial fist while it is elevated.
- Wear an edema glove or other swelling reducing garment as recommended by your occupational therapist.
- Avoid wearing tight clothing or jewelry, or poorly fitting casts or splints.

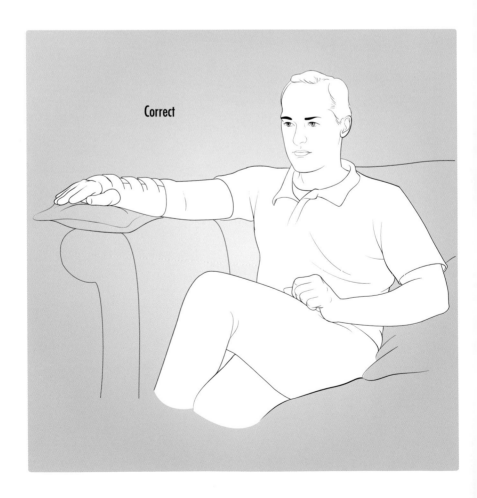

Correct

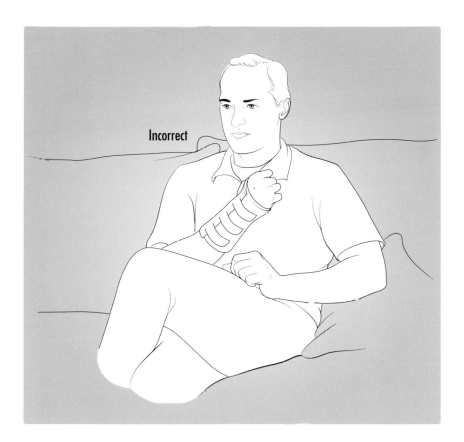

Incorrect

Splint Use

Your doctor and occupational therapist may suggest that you wear a splint to keep your wrist straight in the "neutral" position. Keeping your wrist straight will help control or prevent the symptoms of carpal tunnel syndrome. The splint may be worn while sleeping, driving, or doing specific work activities.

Your occupational therapy practitioner may create a custom-made splint to fit your hand and wrist. The splint will be designed for comfort, function, and purpose.

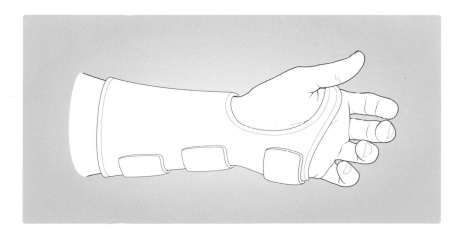

The splint should:

- support your wrist;
- prevent your wrist from bending forward, backward, or sideways;
- allow nearly complete movement of your thumb and fingers;
- allow you to rotate your forearm; and
- allow you to bend your fingers into your palm.

Your doctor or occupational therapist may also suggest that you wear a ready-made splint. He or she will recommend the best splint for you.

Note: Because no two hands are alike, it is best not to choose or use a splint without the advice of your occupational therapist or doctor. It is also best not to borrow a splint from someone else. A pre-made splint or a splint made for someone else may not fit well or may not allow the movement you need to manage carpal tunnel syndrome.

Splint Wear and Care

- Wear only the splint that your occupational therapist or doctor recommends.
- Wear the splint during the recommended times. You may need to wear the splint during the day and at night, or only during the day or night.
- Wear the splint for the recommended length of time. You may need to wear it for several weeks or months. Your occupational therapist or doctor will check it from time to time.
- Clean and maintain your splint as directed by your occupational therapist or occupational therapy assistant.
- Talk with your occupational therapist or occupational therapy assistant if you have questions about wearing your splint.

Use of Adapted or Specially Designed Tools

Adapted or specially designed tools can help prevent or reduce the symptoms of carpal tunnel syndrome. These tools and equipment include items such as:

• tools with larger or built-up handles;
• tools with padded handles;
• ergonomic tools;
• pen or pencil grips; and
• padded, anti-vibration gloves.

Often, everyday items can be adapted for little cost to make them safer and more effective for you. Specially designed tools and assistive devices can also be purchased for specific uses. Your occupational therapist or occupational therapy assistant can suggest adaptations or items that will work best for you.

Exercises

Hand and wrist exercises can be an important part of the treatment plan for carpal tunnel syndrome. Your occupational therapist or doctor will design an exercise program that will give you the greatest benefit.

Keep in mind that no exercise affects everyone the same way. Doing a painful exercise, doing an exercise the wrong way, or not doing a prescribed exercise may cause unneeded problems.

Talk with your occupational therapist or occupational therapy assistant right away if:

• an exercise causes pain;
• you need help learning how to do an exercise; or
• you feel that an exercise is not working well.

Some exercises your occupational therapist or occupational therapy assistant may suggest are shown on pages 26–27. He or she may suggest other ways to do these exercises or may suggest other exercises as well.

Medications

Your doctor may suggest that you take medications to relieve the symptoms of carpal tunnel syndrome. If your doctor does suggest this, be sure to discuss these medications with your doctor.

Surgery

If your symptoms of carpal tunnel syndrome remain after treatment or if your median nerve is badly pinched, your doctor may suggest surgery. Many people with carpal tunnel syndrome do not need surgery, though.

If needed, surgery involves cutting the ligament to relieve pressure on the median nerve. This surgery is usually done without an overnight hospital stay. Your doctor will discuss the method he or she recommends. He or she will also tell you about the surgery's risks and possible complications.

After surgery, your doctor may suggest therapy for a few weeks or as needed. At first, this therapy will include splint management, edema control, and exercises. Later, the therapy will include scar management and more challenging exercises and activities to improve your hand's function, dexterity, and strength. Finally, your doctor and occupational therapist may suggest work on reconditioning and strengthening if needed.

If you used a splint before surgery, your doctor and occupational therapist will want to be sure it still fits correctly. They will also check the splint periodically to clean and maintain it, to prevent pressure sores, and to ensure comfort.

Advice for Daily Activities

Changing the way you do daily activities can help prevent and relieve the symptoms of carpal tunnel syndrome. Your occupational therapist or occupational therapy assistant will help you learn how to make needed changes. He or she will also suggest useful assistive devices or ways to adapt the tools you use.

Keep Your Wrist Straight

When your wrist is straight in the neutral position, the carpal tunnel is at its widest size. This gives the median nerve more room and relieves the pressure on the nerve.

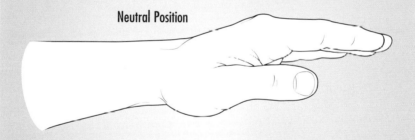

Neutral Position

When you bend your hand forward or backward at the wrist, or when you twist your hand too far to the side, the carpal tunnel narrows and more pressure is placed on the median nerve. This can cause the symptoms of carpal tunnel syndrome.

Wearing a splint, if recommended, and positioning your wrist and hand properly may help prevent or reduce the symptoms of carpal tunnel syndrome.

In general, when doing daily activities, it is important to:

- Keep your wrist straight in the neutral position whenever possible.
- Avoid repeating the same movement over a period of time.
- Take frequent breaks or change tasks often to rest your hand and wrist.
- Avoid flexing, twisting, or bending your wrist, especially into awkward positions.
- Avoid sustained gripping and pinching with your hand or fingers.
- Use your whole hand instead of only one or two fingers and your thumb when grasping objects.

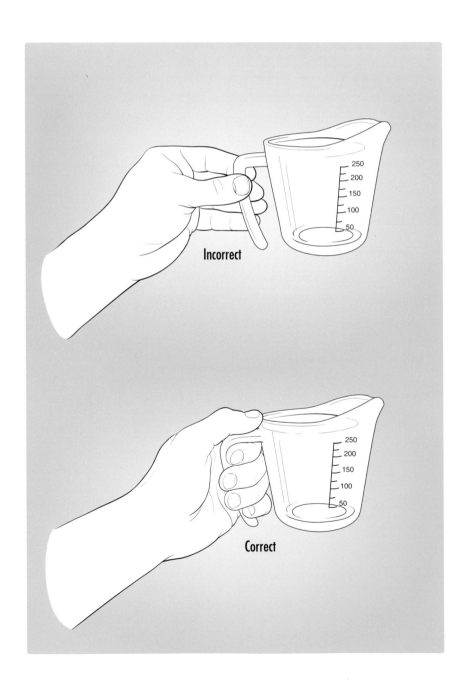

- Use tools that make tasks easier.
- Ask others to help you do tasks that may cause symptoms or make symptoms worse.

Advice for doing some common daily activities is given below. Talk with your occupational therapist or occupational therapy assistant if you have questions about how to do work, household, or leisure activities.

Working at a Computer

- Use an adjustable chair that has wheels but no arm rests.
- Adjust the chair seat height so your elbows and wrists are level with the keyboard. Your elbows should be at your sides and your forearms should be parallel to the floor.
- Adjust the height of the chair back so it supports your spine.
- Place your feet flat on the floor or on a foot rest.
- Place the monitor at eye level, straight in front of you.
- Place typing material at eye level.
- When using a mouse, move your entire arm and shoulder instead of only your hand.
- Use a keyboard that fits your hand size and does not force your wrist to bend up or down or too far to the side.
- When using a laptop computer, attach a separate, larger keyboard that has well-spaced keys.
- Be sure that the keys on your keyboard work properly.
- When not typing, occasionally rest your wrists lightly on a padded wrist rest or a rolled hand towel.
- Change activities often or take frequent breaks to rest your wrists and hands.

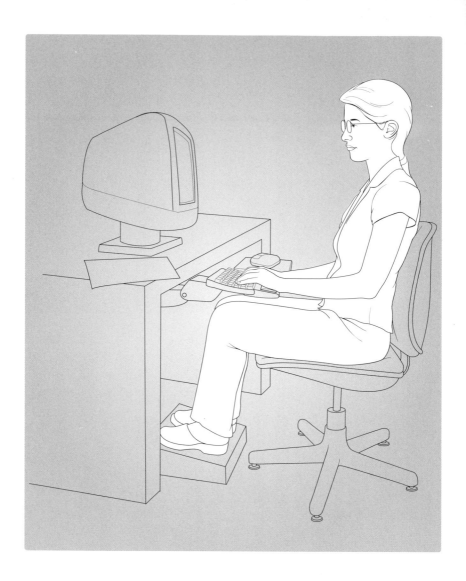

- Adjust the chair height so your elbows and wrists are level with the keyboard and your forearms are parallel to the floor.

- Adjust the chair back to support your spine.

- Keep your feet flat on the floor or on a foot rest.

- Place the monitor at eye level, straight in front of you.

- Place typing material at eye level.

- When not typing, occasionally rest your wrists on a padded wrist rest.

Using Tools

- Keep your wrist straight in the neutral position whenever possible.
- Avoid repetitive tasks and constant gripping of tools over a period of time. Take frequent rest and stretch breaks, or change activities.
- Use two hands or your entire hand and as many fingers as possible to hold the tool.
- Avoid placing excessive force against the heel of your hand. For example, use an automatic electric stapler instead of a manual stapler.

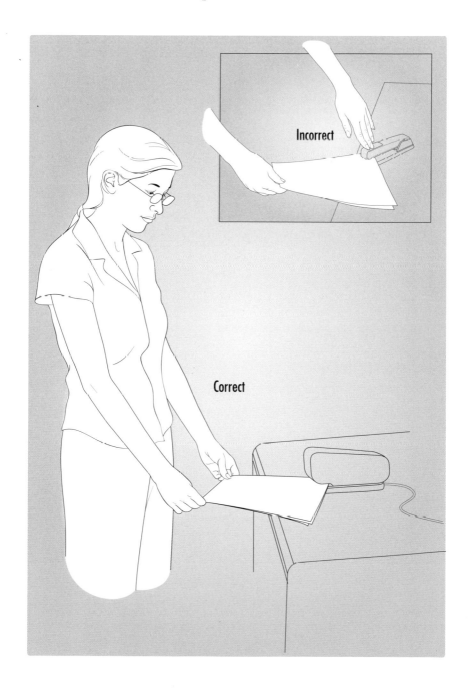

Incorrect

Correct

- Use ergonomic tools or tools with larger, built-up handles. Please refer to the illustration of the ergonomic hammer.
- Avoid using your hand as a hammer.
- Wear anti-vibration gloves (not shown in the picture below) when using vibrating tools such as power sanders, power drills, lawn mowers, and string weed trimmers. When using a power sander, place your palm on top of the sander to distribute the pressure evenly.

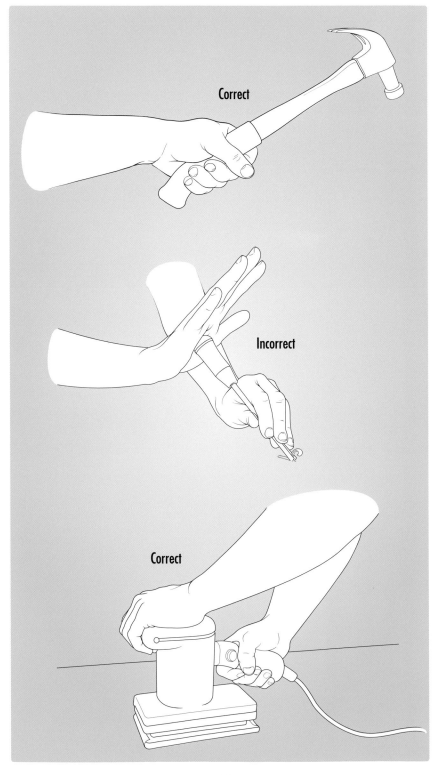

- Use power tools or automated machines whenever possible. When using a power drill, keep your wrist in a neutral position and hold the drill in a straight position.
- Avoid using vibrating tools over periods of time. Take frequent rest and stretch breaks, and rotate job tasks.
- To reduce vibration, keep tools and other equipment in good working order.

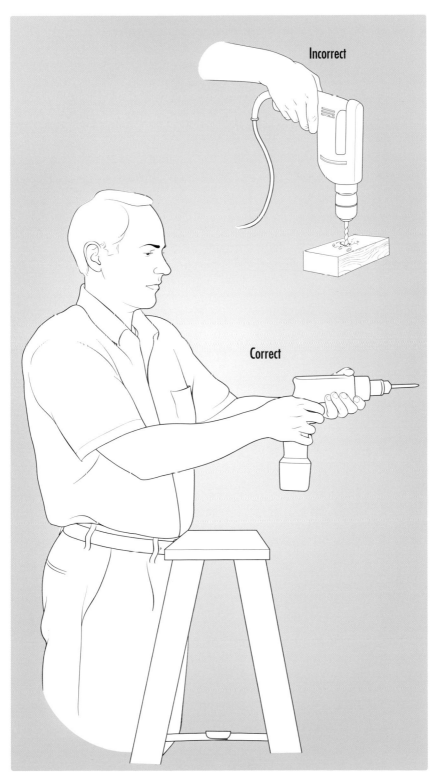

Working Around Your Home

- Try to keep your wrist straight in a neutral position when doing household tasks.
- Change hands often when doing tasks such as vacuuming or dusting.
- To carry small items, place them in a basket and carry the basket on your forearm rather than in your hand.
- Change activities or take frequent breaks to rest your hand and wrist.
- Avoid gripping or pinching items over a period of time.

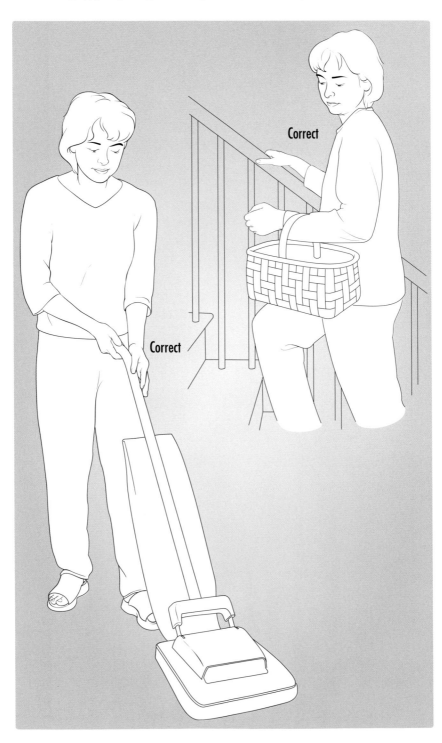

Preparing and Eating Meals

- Lift and carry trays, pots, pans, and bowls with your palms on the bottom, rather than gripping or pinching the sides. Use both hands.
- Use an electric can opener instead of a manual can opener.
- Use a jar opener instead of your hands.
- Use lightweight pots, pans, and serving dishes.
- Open packages with scissors rather than your hands.
- When making large meals, break the tasks into steps and do some steps ahead of time.
- Choose foods that can be prepared without using repetitive motions.
- Ask others for help with tasks that may make your symptoms worse.
- When grocery shopping, use a cart instead of carrying a basket.
- Buy smaller sizes that are easier to handle and carry.
- Buy items in easy-to-open packages.

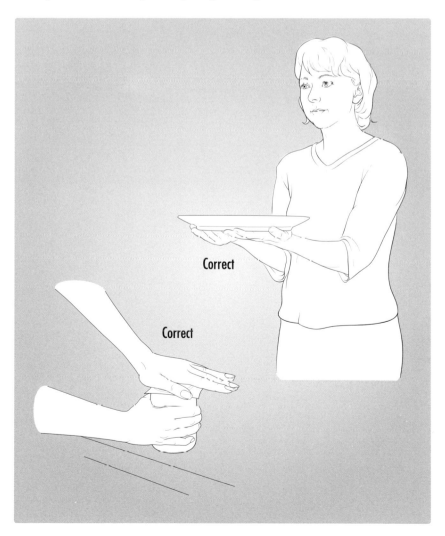

Correct

Correct

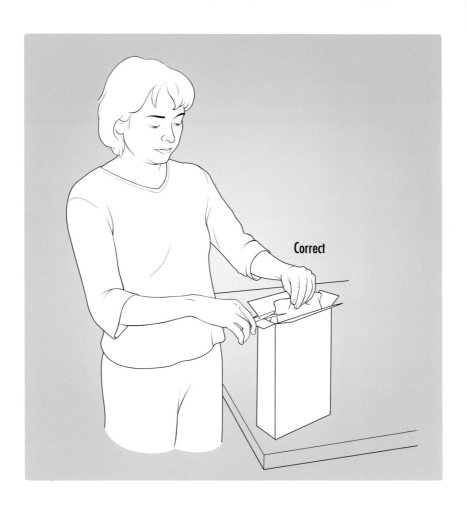

Correct

Writing

- Grip the pen loosely and use a flowing motion.
- Choose a pen that flows well.
- Use a thick pen or pencil, or build up the size using a foam or triangular grip.
- Make photocopies instead of pressing hard to make multiple "carbon" copies.

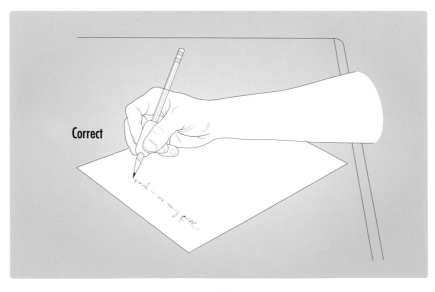

Correct

Sleeping

- Keep your wrist straight in a neutral position when sleeping.
- Wear a splint when sleeping, if recommended.
- Place your hand and forearm on a pillow for comfort and easier positioning.

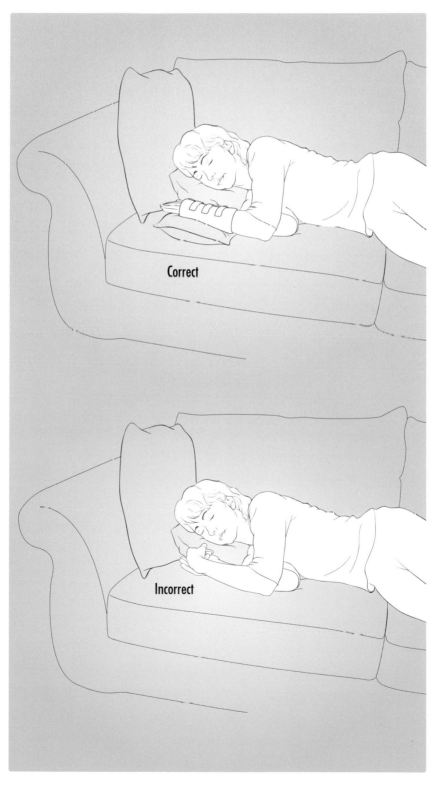

Correct

Incorrect

Driving

- Keep your wrist straight in a neutral position when holding the steering wheel.

- Avoid clenching the steering wheel for periods of time. Relax and hold the wheel firmly but comfortably.

- Consider using an enlarged or padded steering wheel cover.

- If the steering wheel vibrates, have the alignment of your tires checked and corrected.

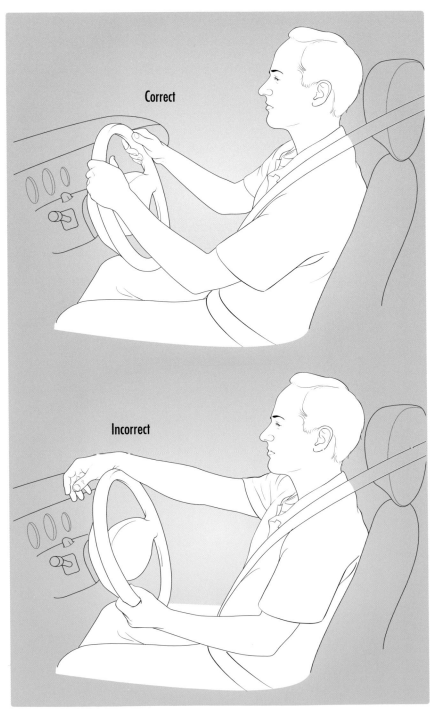

Correct

Incorrect

Leisure Activities

- Avoid leisure activities that involve repetitive use of your hand or wrist.

- Avoid leisure activities that involve sustained gripping or pinching.

- Take frequent breaks or change tasks often to rest your hand and wrist.

- Reduce, modify, or stop doing leisure activities that may make your symptoms worse.

- If you are not able to do an activity you enjoy, find a new activity to replace it.

- Talk with your occupational therapist and occupational therapy assistant about ways to modify your leisure activities.

Helpful Exercises

Exercises can benefit people with carpal tunnel syndrome. Your occupational therapist or doctor will design an individualized exercise program to give you the greatest benefit.

The exercises suggested here are effective for many people. Talk with your occupational therapist or occupational therapy assistant about including these exercises in your treatment program.

Your occupational therapist or occupational therapy assistant will tell you how long to hold each position and how many times to do the exercises. Do not squeeze a ball while doing hand exercises because this can make your symptoms worse.

If an exercise causes pain or if you are unsure how to do an exercise, stop doing it and talk with your occupational therapist or doctor.

Tendon Gliding Exercises

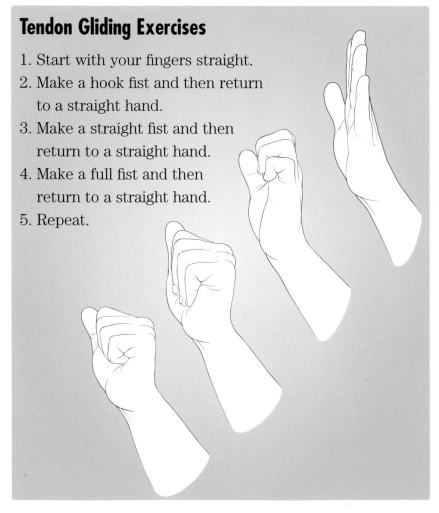

1. Start with your fingers straight.
2. Make a hook fist and then return to a straight hand.
3. Make a straight fist and then return to a straight hand.
4. Make a full fist and then return to a straight hand.
5. Repeat.

Median Nerve Gliding Exercises at the Wrist

1. Begin by making a fist, with your wrist in the neutral position.
2. Straighten your fingers and thumb.
3. Bend your wrist back and move your thumb away from your palm.

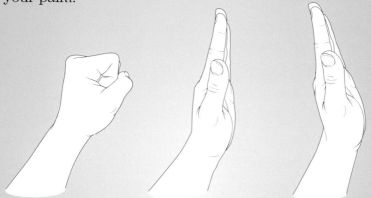

4. Turn your wrist palm up.
5. Use your other hand to gently pull your thumb farther away from your palm in the direction of the arrow.

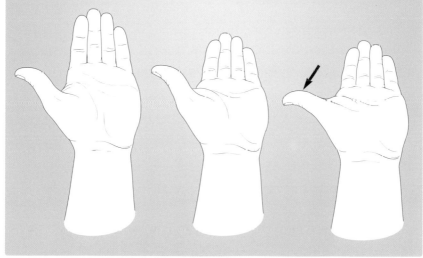

Wrist Exercises

1. With your fingers bent into a "hook," gently extend your wrist by bending it backward.
2. Release your fingers from the hook.
3. Gently flex your wrist forward.

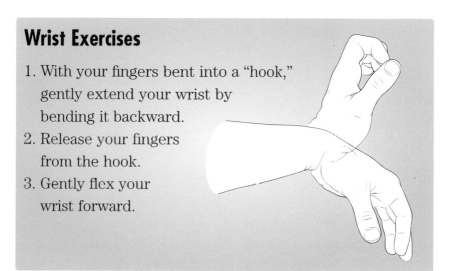

Your Treatment Program

Ask your occupational therapist to fill in the following information about your treatment program.

General Precautions

- Keep your wrist straight in the neutral position whenever possible.
- Avoid flexing, twisting, or bending your wrist.
- Avoid sustained gripping and pinching with your hand or fingers.
- Take frequent breaks or change tasks often to rest your hand and wrist.
- Avoid repeating the same movement over a period of time.
- To grasp objects, use your whole hand instead of only one or two fingers and your thumb.

Edema (Swelling) Management

- Elevate your hand: _____
- When elevating your hand, keep your hand above your elbow and keep your elbow above your shoulder.
- Comfortably open and close your hand into a comfortable fist or partial fist while it is elevated.
- Use an edema glove as recommended by your occupational therapy practitioner:_____
- Avoid wearing tight clothing or jewelry.

Splint Use

Wear your splint(s) while:

- Sleeping

- Driving

- _____

- _____

Wear your splint(s) no more than:

_____

How to clean your splint(s):_____

_____

_____

_____

Skin care precautions: _____

_____

_____

_____

Heat sensitivity precautions (for custom-made splints):

_____

_____

_____

_____

Adapted/Specially Designed Tool Recommendations

• Tool: _____   _____

   Use:_____

   _____

• Tool: _____

   Use:_____

   _____

• Tool: _____   _____

   Use:_____

   _____

• Tool: _____

   Use:_____

   _____

Exercises

- Tendon gliding:_____

_____

_____

_____

- Median nerve gliding:_____

_____

_____

_____

- Wrist exercises:_____

_____

_____

_____

- Other:_____

_____

_____

_____

_____

_____

_____

_____

_____

_____

_____

_____

_____

_____

Equipment Information

Occupational Therapy

Occupational therapy is the profession dedicated to helping individuals regain their ability to function more productively in their communities, at schools, at work, and at home. Occupational therapy helps us master the skills we need in our everyday lives. These skills include eating, dressing, taking care of personal hygiene, driving, working, going to school, and managing personal, household, and financial affairs.

The Role of Occupational Therapy

The skills of a knowledgeable health care specialist are needed when health problems challenge a person's ability to engage in daily life.

Occupational therapists help a wide variety of people, including those who have limitations following a stroke or heart attack and individuals who have arthritis and Alzheimer's. They help people who have received broken bones or other injuries from falls. Occupational therapists also can help individuals who have vision or cognitive problems that threaten their ability to drive.

The American Occupational Therapy Association

The American Occupational Therapy Association (AOTA) represents the professionals who have chosen this valuable health care career. Founded in 1917, the American Occupational Therapy Association has played a key role in meeting the health care needs of our nation.

The name of the profession originated in the early twentieth century when progressive thinkers in health care advanced the belief that those patients who engaged in "purposeful occupations" such as crafts and practical work activities experienced a more successful recovery.

Throughout the twentieth century, occupational therapy met the needs of returning veterans, polio survivors, people with mental illness, and people with physical disabilities.

Today, occupational therapy is a vibrant, dynamic profession that helps people of all ages lead better lives in the face of health challenges.

The National Office of AOTA is located at:
4720 Montgomery Lane
Bethesda, Maryland 20824-1220.

The Association may be reached at 301-652-AOTA (2682).
The TDD is 800-377-8555, and the fax number is 301-652-7711.
Go to AOTA's Web site at www.aota.org for more information on AOTA or occupational therapy.

To order additional copies of this consumer guide, or to learn about AOTA's other publications, please visit our Web site at www.aota.org and click on the Online Store, or call toll free 877-404-AOTA (2682).

DATE DUE
